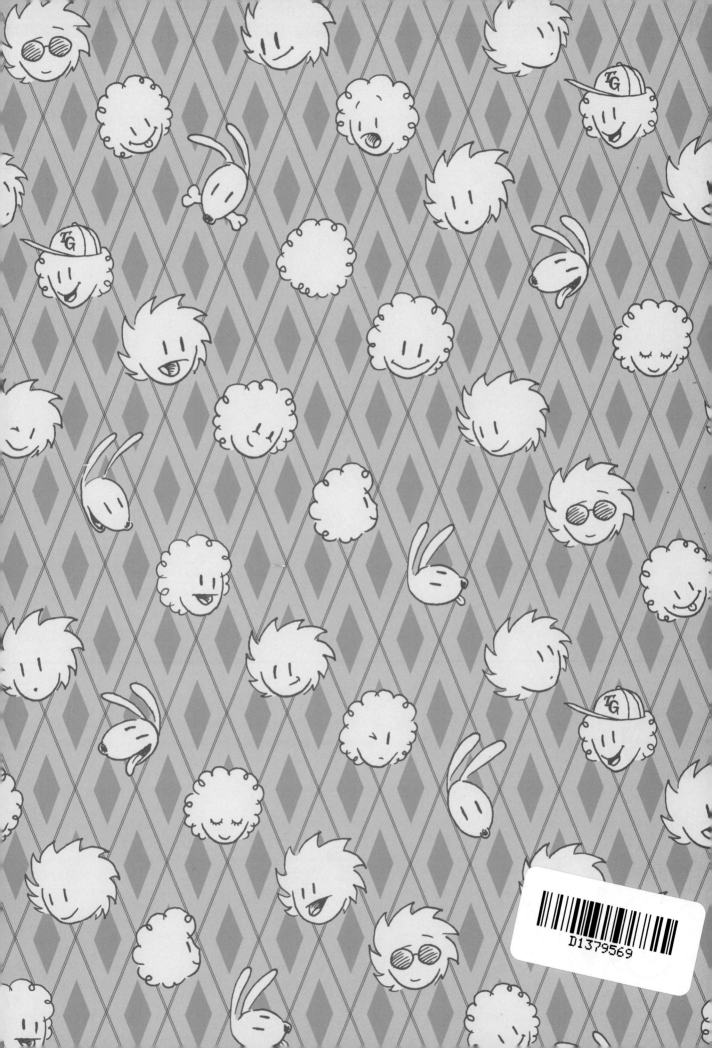

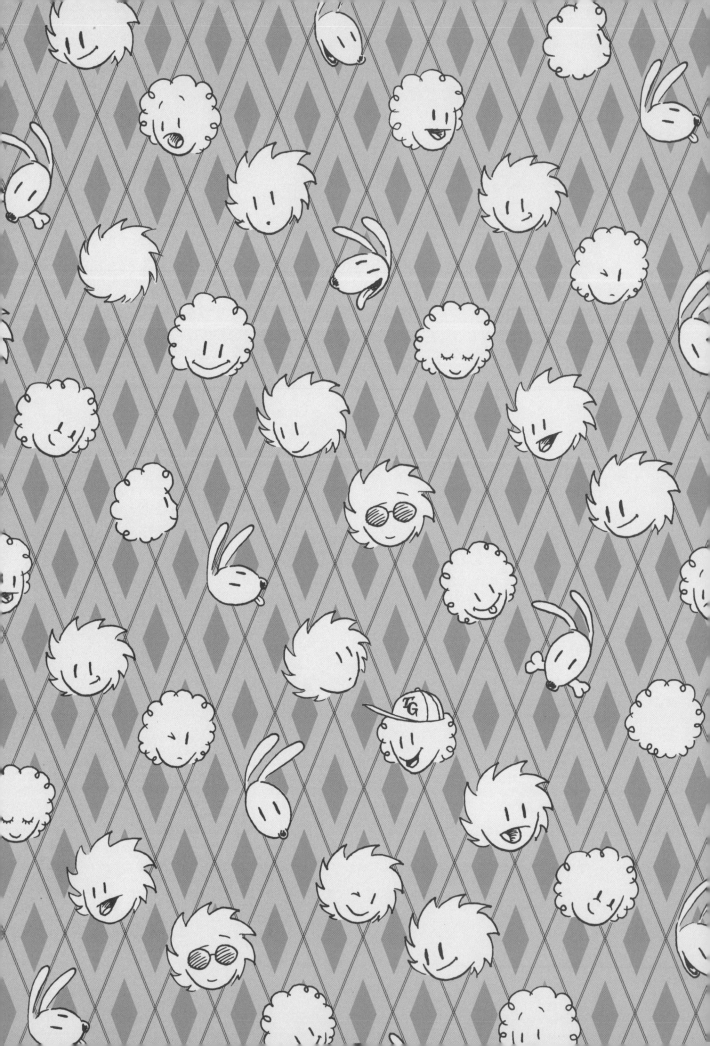

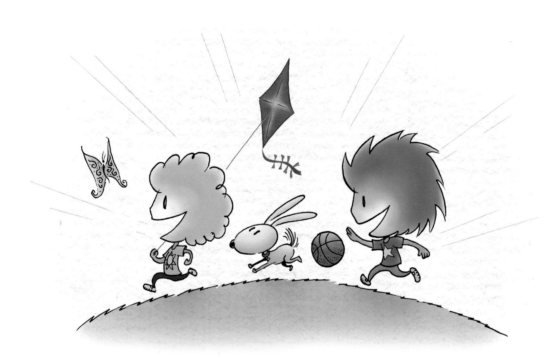

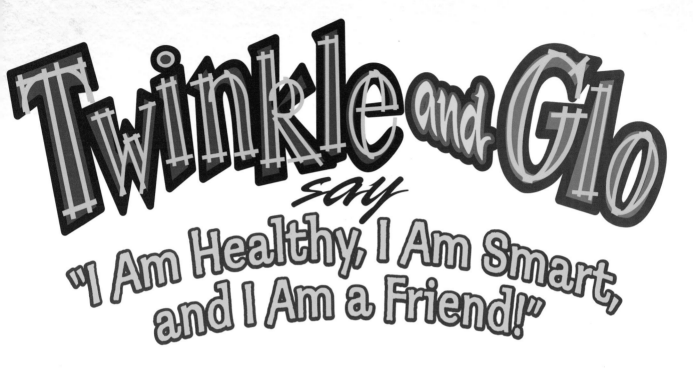

Twinkle and Glo say "I Am Healthy, I Am Smart, and I Am a Friend!"

CONCEIVED AND COMPILED BY

JUDY JOSEPH, MLS

DRAWN BY

SCOTT JOHNSON AND STEPHANIE BALL

CONTRIBUTORS

DEAN PRINA, MD   ELIZABETH LOESCHER, MA

VERNITA VALLEZ, PHD   JESSICA BASS MCCOY, MA

LAURA PRITCHETT, PHD

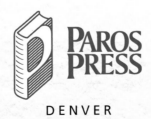

PAROS PRESS

DENVER

For information, contact
Paros Press
1551 Larimer Street, Suite 1301
Denver, CO 80202
303-893-3331

www.parospress.com

LCCN 2010937045

ISBN 978-0-9702093-8-2

Printed in Canada
1 3 5 7 9 10 8 6 4 2

Good morning, good morning! It's time to arise
and learn to be healthy, friendly and wise.

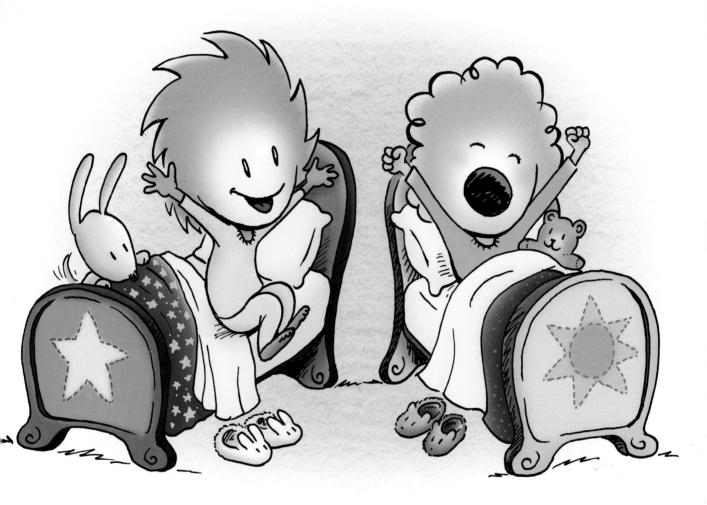

You are special, you are *you*,
and there are good things that we can do.
Yes, oh yes, there are things I will say
as we jump and we skip through this colorful day.
Twinkle says let's make every day special and grand!
So, get up, get up, Glo, and give me your hand!

Wake up with a smile, wake up being giggly,
wake up being merry and joyfully wiggly!
Each day is special, especially for you,
A day full of moments to try something new!

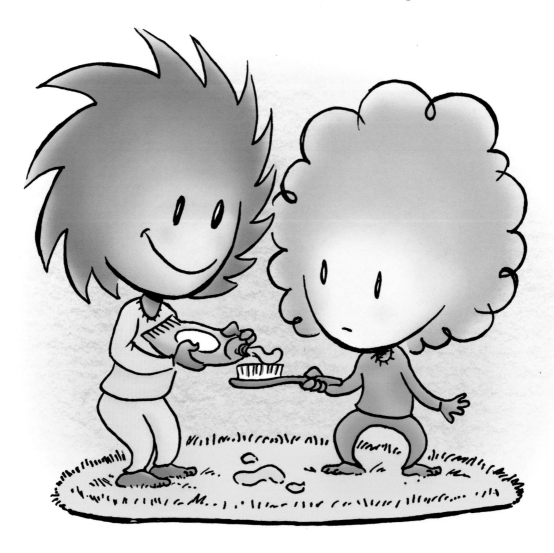

First, start the day right
with a smile that's bright.
Brushing your teeth
makes them fresh and so white.

Climb on up, have a seat for a good breakfast treat.
Let's have something yummy to drink and to eat!

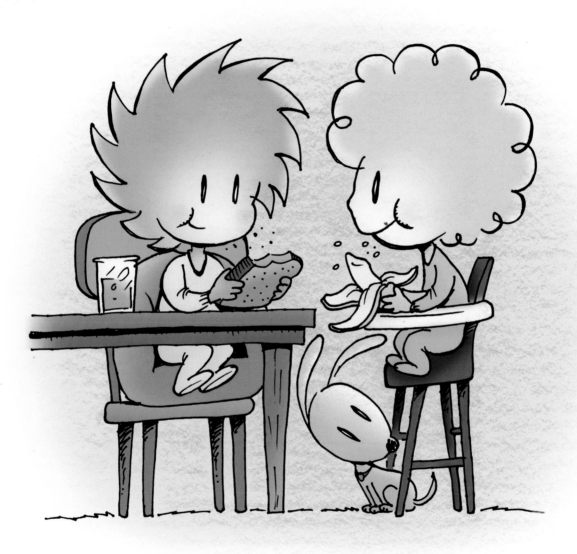

What you put in your body really does matter,
so not just potato chips, soda, and cake batter!
Take care of your body, oh please oh please!
Eat fruits and veggies, bread and cheese.

What should we do? What should we do?
Sit and watch TV? No, no, let's do something new!

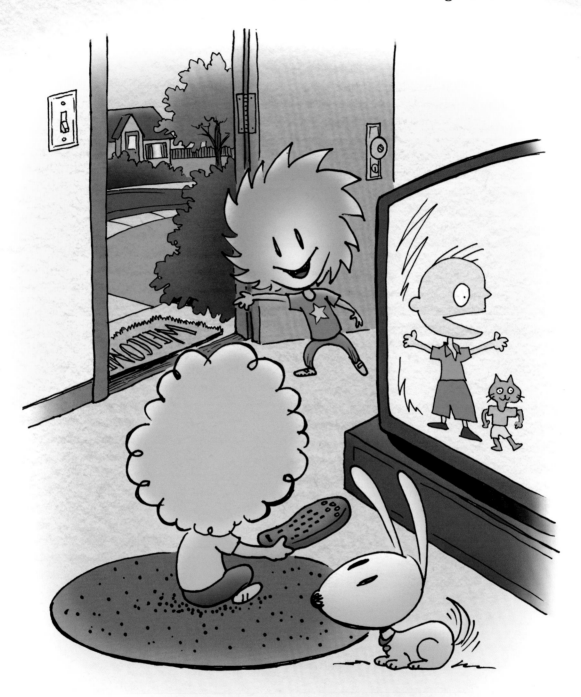

The sun is out, it's shining bright,
Let's go have fun with all of our might.
Yes indeed, it's a very nice day.
Yes, oh yes, let's go out and play.

Look! Look! A new family is just moving in!
Let's go over and make a new friend!

Say our names,
Play some games,
Look our new friends in the eye.
Try hard not to be shy!

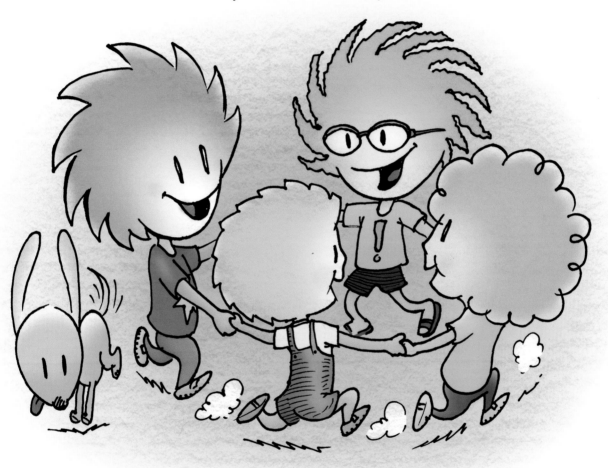

Friends are friends no matter the weather.
Friends are people who make our lives better.
Your newest friend is the one you didn't even know
When you said hello a few minutes ago.

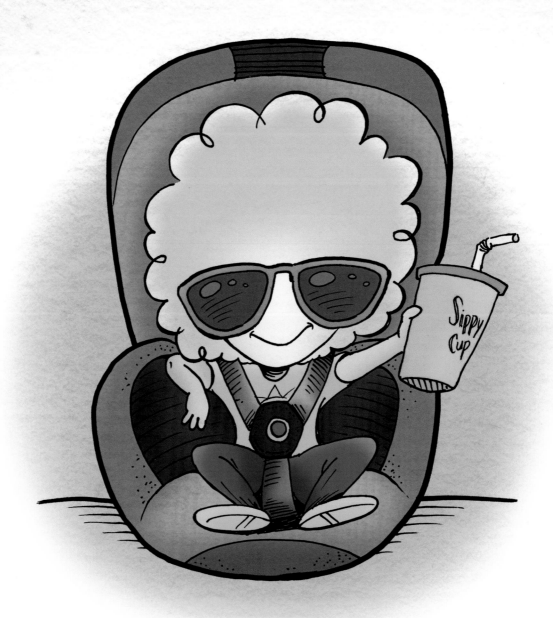

Now it's time to go for a ride.
Hop in your carseat when you get inside.
Pull that seatbelt across your lap —
pull it real tight and attach with a SNAP!

When we get out
We MUST look about.

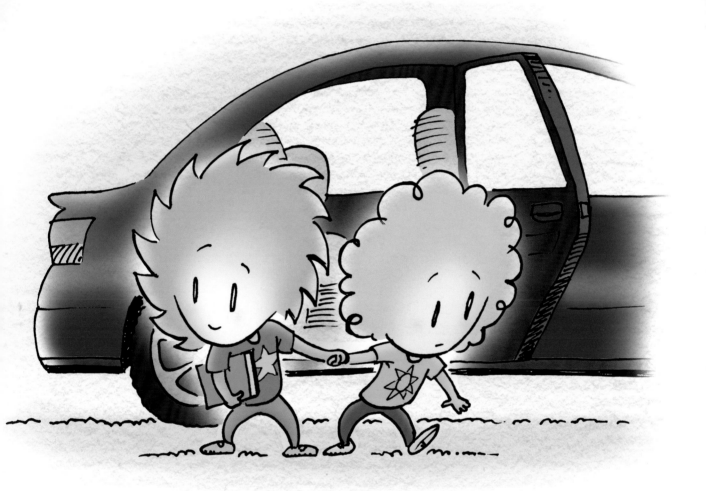

Take hold of a hand, look left and look right,
Watch out for traffic and wait for the light.
Look out for bicycles, dumptrucks and cars
and anything else that could make you see stars!

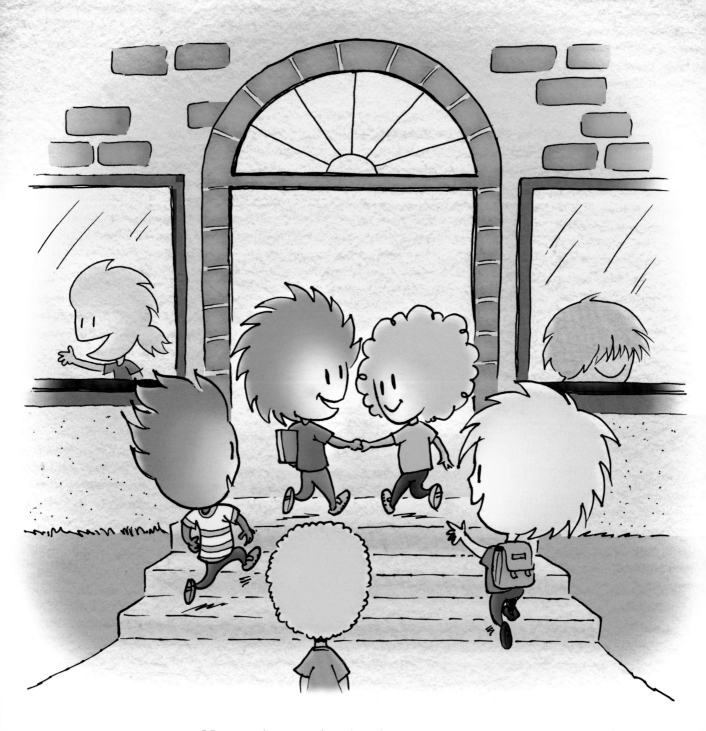

Now we're at school (which is so very cool)
where our friends are the best and the teachers all rule!
It's a very neat place for us children to learn,
where our minds whirl, twirl and turn.

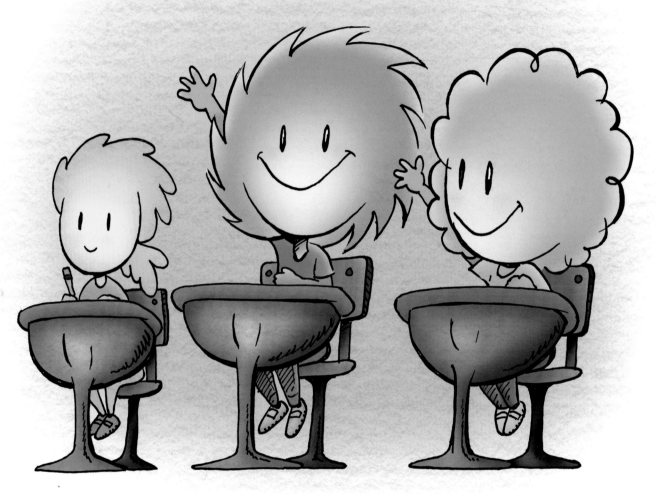

Curious minds are open and bright.
Asking questions is how we get things right.
If you don't know something, don't sit and boo-hoo!
Just ask a question! Like *what? when? why? who?*

Remember this: It's up to YOU to learn!
(But raise your hand and wait for your turn.)

Think about new words you find,
Try to keep them inside your mind.
Write them down...
Whisper a sound...

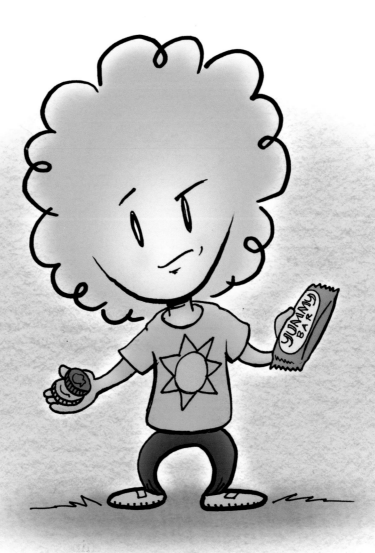

Even practicing math will come in so handy
when you're counting your change and buying some candy.
Numbers can be such a wonderful deal
for building or saving or cooking a meal!

It is lunchtime now and our tummies are rumbly
But before you eat — and don't get grumbly! —
You have to stop and wash your hands.
They are covered with dirt and sand!
And even though germs are tiny and small
They can make you so sick, so get rid of them all!

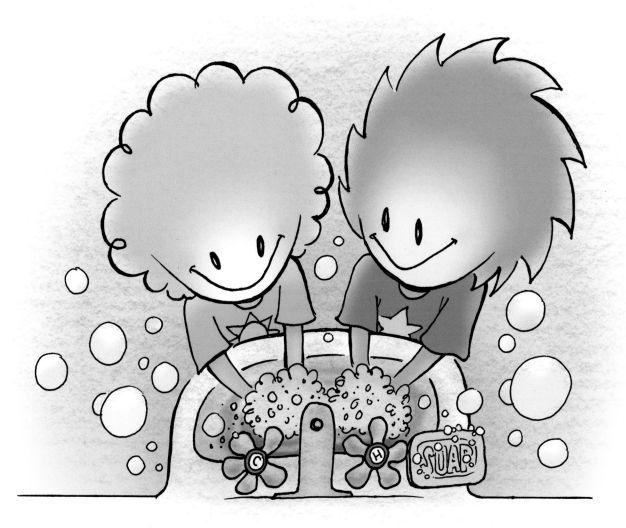

It's easy to forget, but you should not.
Wash your hands with soap and rub them a lot!
(Because, you know, it's not fun having snot.)

Did I say it before? Well, I'll say it again!
The food you pick can help you win
Races and hopscotch and everything fun
And make you as bright as the afternoon sun.

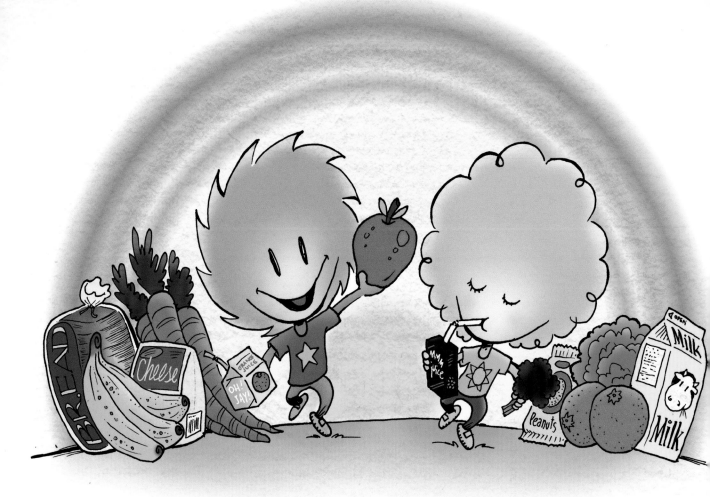

Now that our lunchtime is finally here,
Remember fruits and veggies are nothing to fear.
Choose and think and think and choose –
Eat every color of the rainbow, even the blues!
A glass of cold milk is important, too.
Soy or cow, either will do!

Now it's recess and time to play.
What's this? What do you say?

MY WAY! MY WAY!
OR ELSE I WILL NOT PLAY!

Well! That is not a nice thing to say!

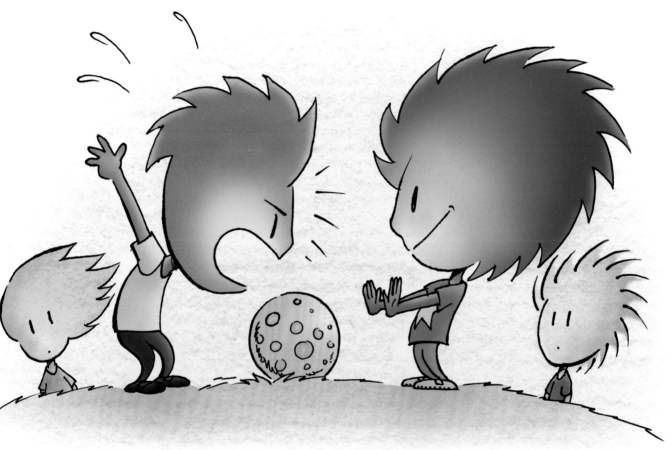

Let's work it out.
Let's not shout.
Please, oh please, do not pout!!
Instead, say nicely:

But we did it your way yesterday!
Let's let someone else choose today!

Sometimes it's hard not to fight.
Take a breath, be polite.
Everyone can win a little
If we meet in the middle.

When another child starts a fight,
Always remember what's wrong and what's right.
Listen first.
Mean words make it worse.

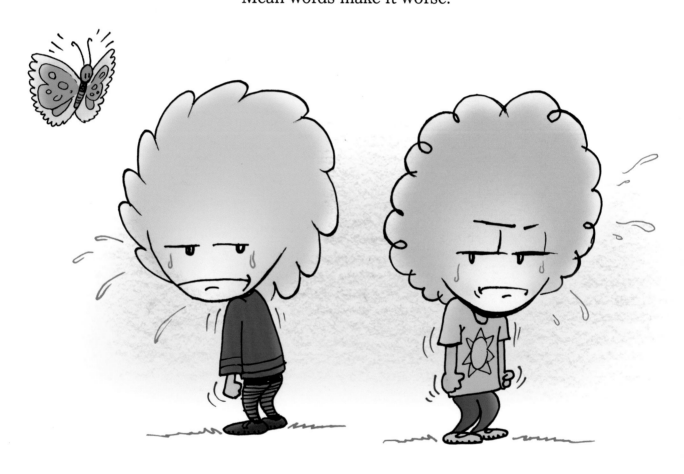

If you're feeling angry and hot,
Take three breaths and take a short walk.
Telling someone how you feel is one thing to do.
Choose how you act — don't let bad feelings control *you*.

Sometimes it seems like the whole world is wrong.
You can't get what you want and you don't feel so strong.
But it's okay to cry! It's okay to be sad!
That's all part of living, to not always be glad!

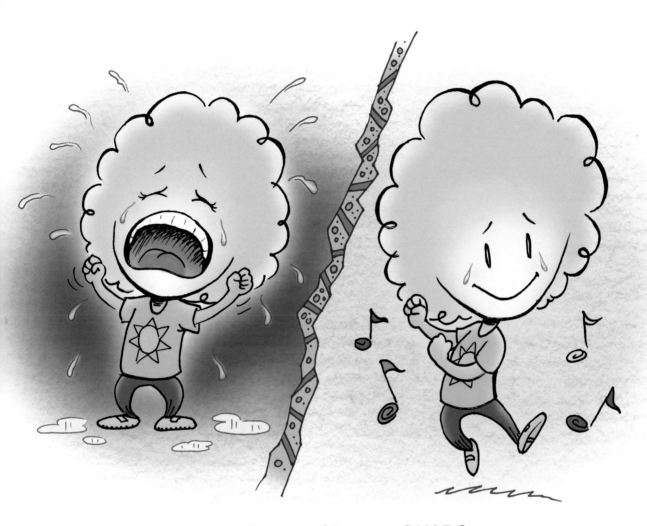

But there are things you CAN DO
When you feel sad and blue.
You can draw, or sing, or dance,
Or wiggle about in a silly prance!
Get a friend to go along —
You'll feel better before long.

Remember, when we're sick, do not go out.
We stay in our home and we don't roam about.
In our own little bed, we can sneeze, sneeze and sneeze.
But use some tissues, if you please!

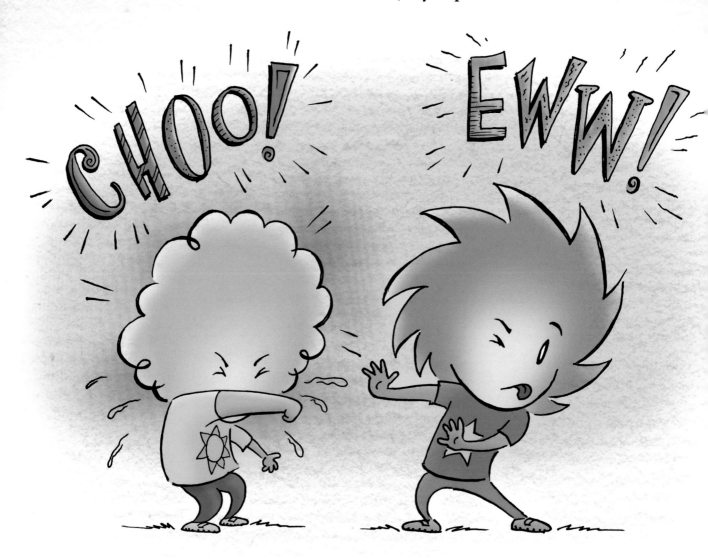

We cannot just spread nasty germs all around,
not all over school, or all over town.
That's why I say: don't leave home if you're sick.
Isn't it smarter to get better quick?
Stay home, I say, and quietly play.
For yourself and your health, stay home for a day.

Now let's go out
To play about,
Remember to move every day.
Get up, go out, go play!

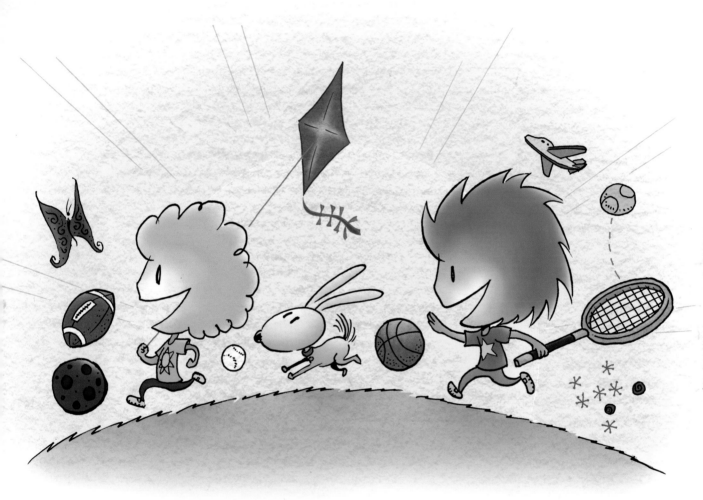

Ride a bike.
Fly a kite.
Soccer, hockey, basketball
(Oh yes, you can play them all).
Play alone — or play on a team.
Jump up and down and scream and scream!

If you don't want your head to be cracked,
Use a helmet — that's a fact!
Bones can break,
Skin can scrape.
Being careful is up to you.
I say this because it's so true.

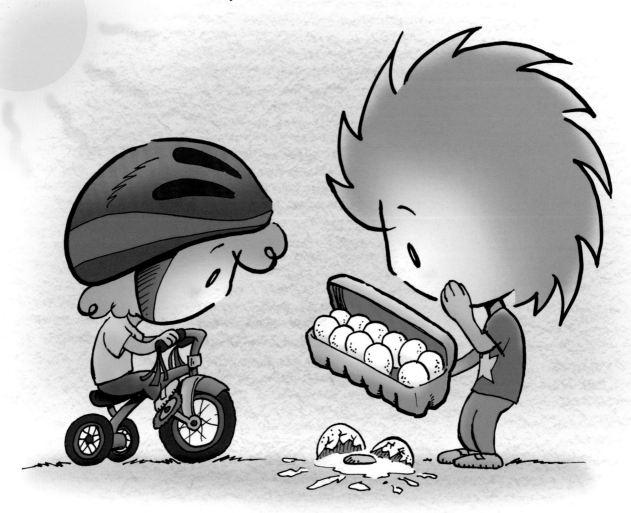

But danger can also be very quiet.
It's not always a big ruckusy-riot.
Even the sun can hurt you, too,
So putting on sunscreen is a good thing to do.

Danger! Danger!
What's going on?
I feel hot, or cold,
Or something feels wrong.
Well! That's the time to look for some help.
You don't have to be by yourself!

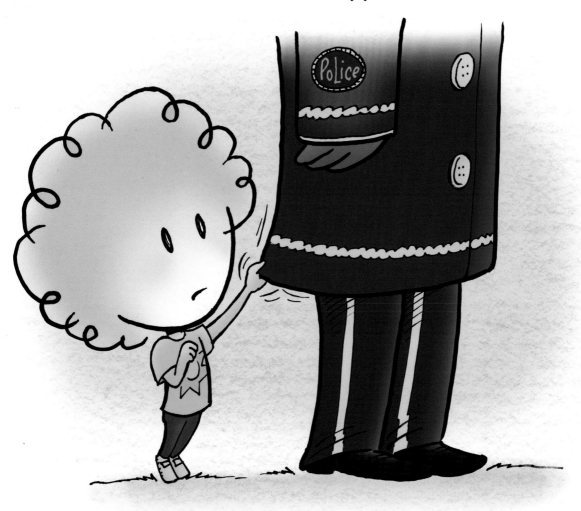

Tell an adult if you see a bully be mean
Or guns anywhere — they shouldn't be seen!
If a stranger gives you candy and says "Let's go!"
Run away fast and say "NO NO NO!"
And if it's a fire you see or you smell,
Go tell an adult so that all can be well.

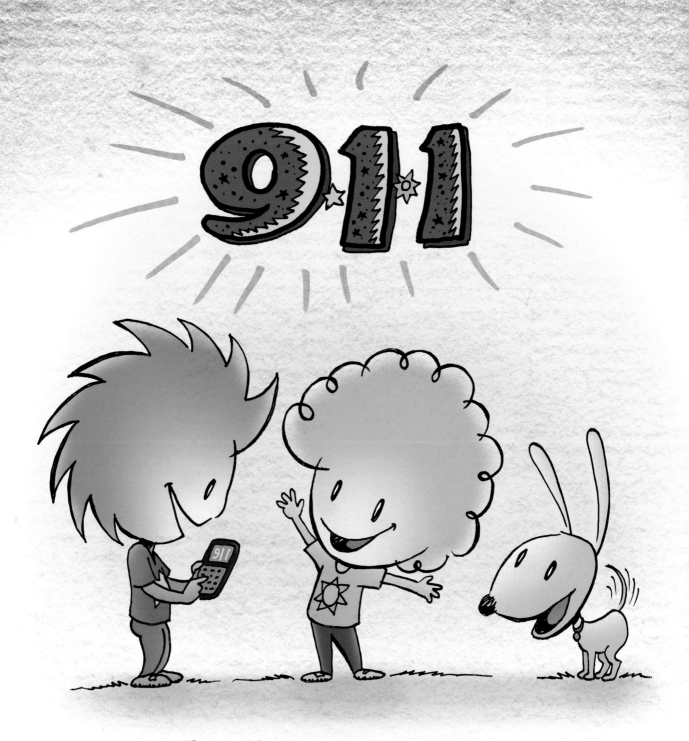

911

If an accident happens, don't turn and flee.
Learn "9-1-1" by the time you are three!
Tell them the problem, and try not to shout.
Someone will come and they'll help you out.
Just say where you are and just what you need.
Stay calm and someone will be there with speed!

Now it's time for us to go home, that's right!
There's no better place to be polite.
Say "please" and "thank you" and mean what you say
And do this every single day.
Be nice to grandparents and neighbors, too,
And pets and creatures — oh please, oh do!

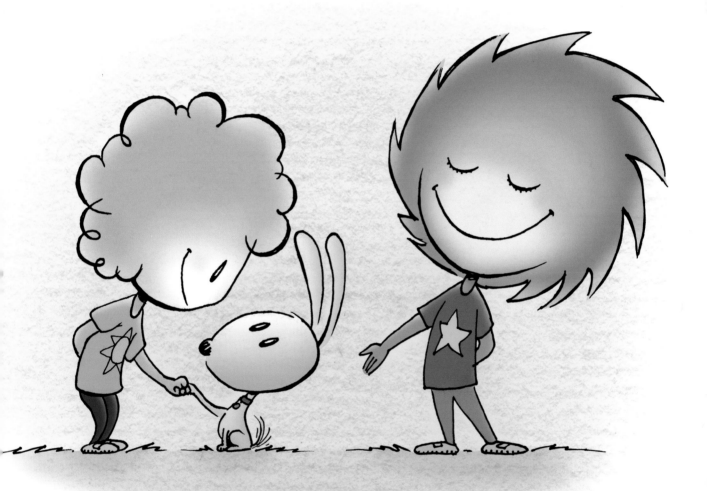

There are many things to learn, oh my.
It's sometimes hard, and it means you must try.
But it can make a big difference, to be healthy and smart,
If you only learn how to do your part.

The day has been long, the day has been fine.
Time to settle in body and mind.
A yoga stretch, a calm breathing place,
A moment or two to create your own space.

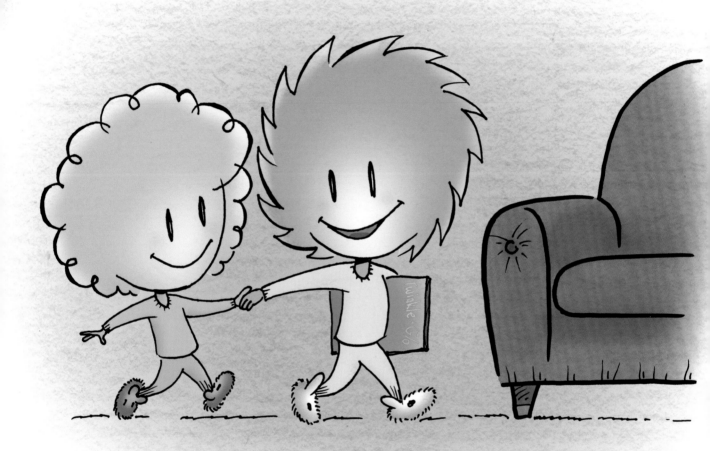

A bath, a snuggle, a so-happy time,
A warm lullaby or a sweet whispered rhyme.
A time to be grateful for the day that you've had,
Since life is so special and makes you so glad.

Now take a rest from thinking so hard
From all the thoughts and being on guard.
Curl up with a book from the library shelf
And imagine such things we can't see for ourself.

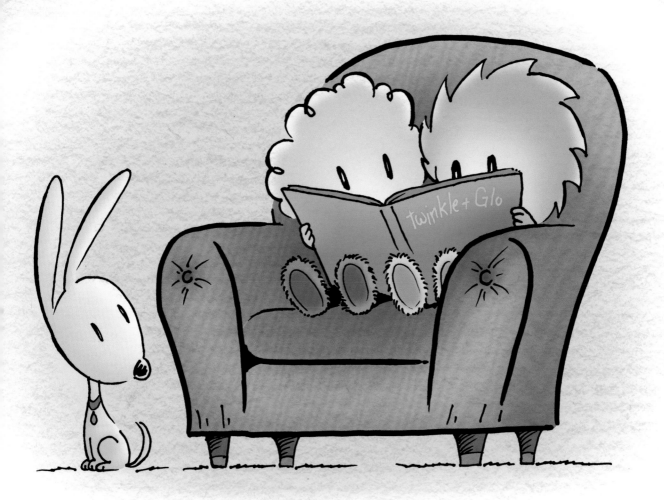

Reading books is a favorite thing —
Horses that fly and dragons that sing.
The more you read, the happier you'll be.
Reading really sets your heart and mind free.

There's lots to remember for every day.
Eat right, be safe, know the right things to say.
This day has been fun, this day has been full,
This day has been totally, awesomely cool!

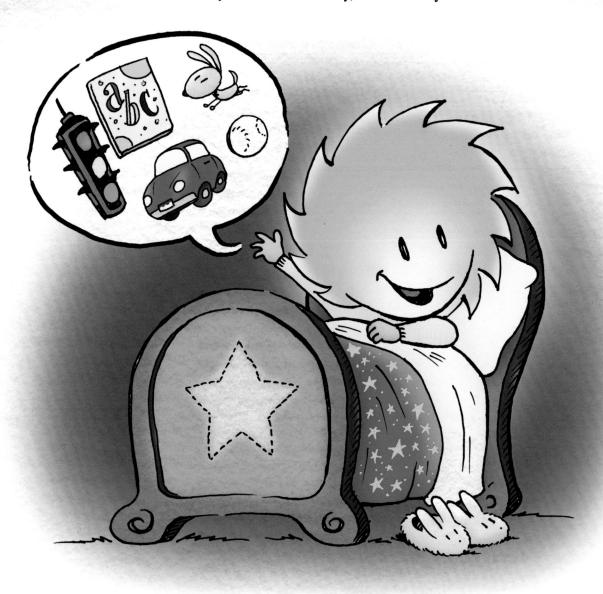

Living well and safe and true
Takes a little bit of work, but it's oh so fun, too.
We both should live well and be smart and kind
And be our best in body and mind.

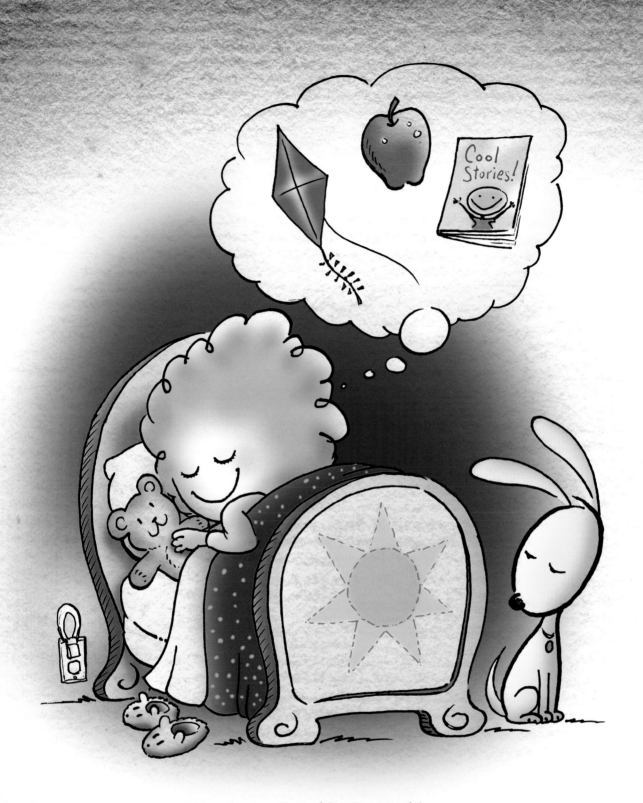

Thank you, Twinkle, for teaching me
There's so much to know and so much to see.
Sweet dreams, Glo! Sweet dreams and good night.
Smile and snuggle and turn off the light.

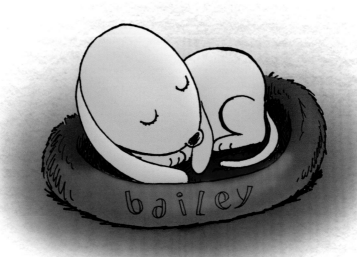

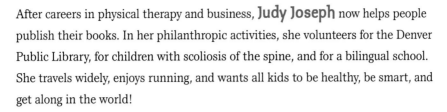

Twinkle and Glo's friends

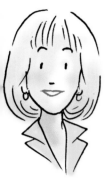

After careers in physical therapy and business, **Judy Joseph** now helps people publish their books. In her philanthropic activities, she volunteers for the Denver Public Library, for children with scoliosis of the spine, and for a bilingual school. She travels widely, enjoys running, and wants all kids to be healthy, be smart, and get along in the world!

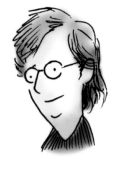

Scott Johnson is a Denver cartoonist, graphic designer and swing musician, with a wife and a daughter who have both come to pretty much accept him for what he is. He's also the author and illustrator of *Little Chrissie Kringle and Other Christmas Cacophony.*

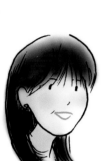

Stephanie Ball is a graphic designer and student at Western State College in Gunnison, Colorado. She's about to receive her Bachelor of Fine Arts in Design, if skiing and snowboarding don't divert her too radically from that pesky classwork.

A pediatrician in private practice with Partners in Pediatrics in Denver, **Dean Prina** is the co-author of *Naturally Healthy Kids,* a book which integrates conventional and holistic treatments for common illnesses of children. Dean received his medical degree from Stanford University, as well as undergraduate degrees in art history and human biology.

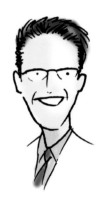

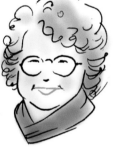
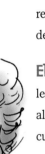

Elizabeth Loescher is an educator, parent, author of five books, and national lecturer on conflict and anger management. She is a pioneer in the field of alternative dispute resolution, having founded The Conflict Center in Denver. Liz is currently the Executive Director of the Georgia Conflict Center in Athens, Georgia.

Vernita Vallez fell in love with books and learning when she had her grandmother as her first grade teacher. She was principal of Escuela de Guadalupe in Denver, and is currently principal of a dual language school in Chicago. She and her husband have finished playing in the mud, building their earth bag house in the Colorado mountains.

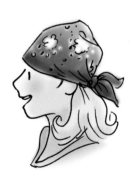

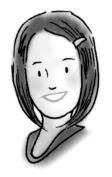

A first grade teacher at Denver's Lowry Elementary, **Jessica Bass McCoy** has written and published two illustrated children's books—*Do You Know What Teachers Really Do After School?* and *Do You Know What Really Happens In The Teacher's Lounge?* Jessica lives in Denver with her husband and her dog Max.

Laura Pritchett is the author/editor of five books for adults, but really had a blast writing this one for children. She lives in northern Colorado with her husband and two kids. She holds a Ph.D. in Literature from Purdue University and teaches at writing workshops around the country. You can find her at www.laurapritchett.com.

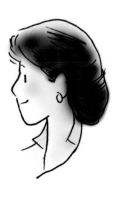

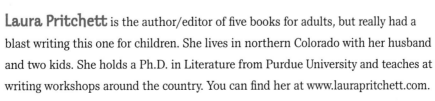
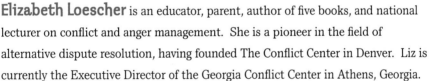

In a light-hearted and loving way,
Twinkle & Glo teach young children important lessons about

Health and Safety

Literacy, Learning and School

Getting Along and Conflict Resolution.

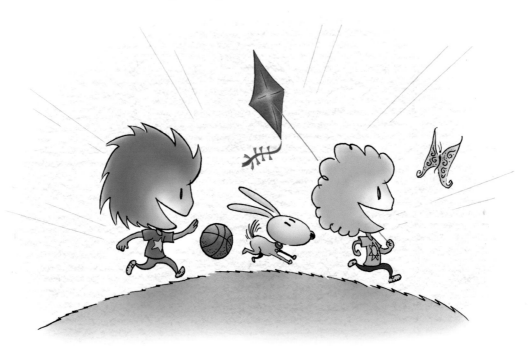

This book is distributed free to 5-year-olds, and all sales profits
benefit children's health, literacy and community building.

For ordering, fundraising opportunities or more information contact:
Paros Press LLC
1551 Larimer St., Suite 1301   Denver CO 80202
303-893-3331   twinkle@parospress.com

www.parospress.com
www.twinkleandglo.org